Nurse Pharmacology C[

A Relaxed Study Guide for the NCLEX Exam

Volume 1: Cardiovascular Medications

Get a FREE set of pharmacology FLASHCARDS

and be the FIRST to know about NEW releases!

Sign up today at:

www.nursereadinessacademy.com

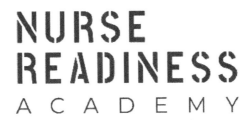

NURSE READINESS A C A D E M Y

ISBN: 9798386729745

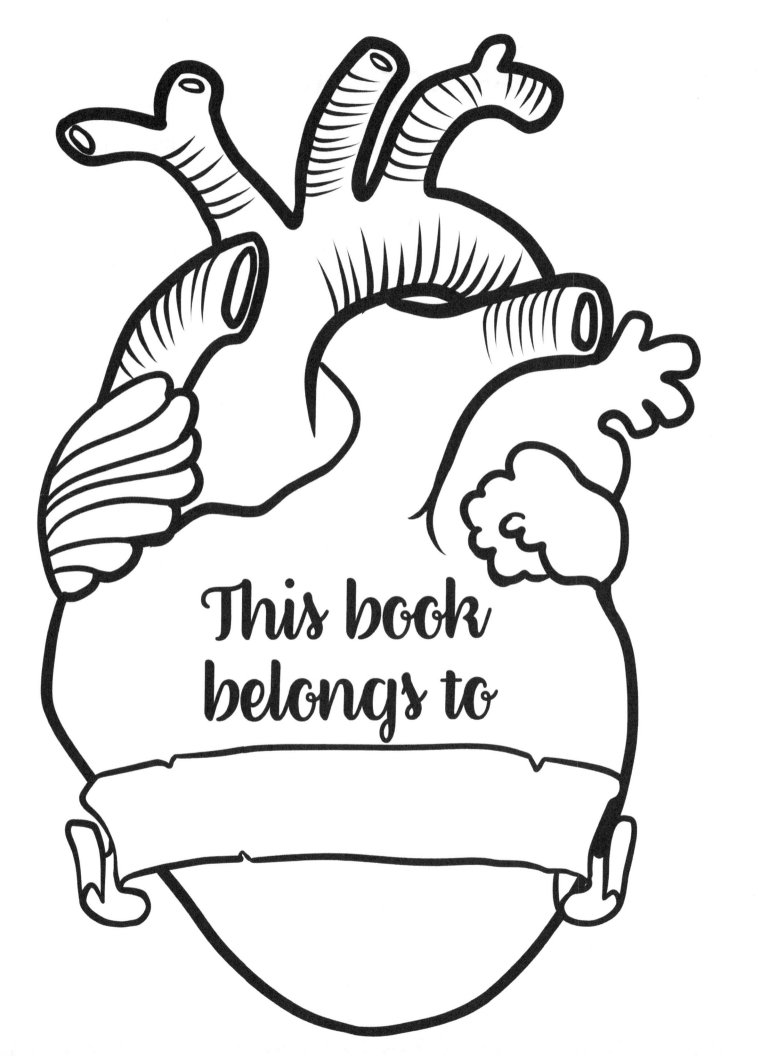

This book
belongs to

TABLE OF CONTENTS

This book covers the following medications in alphabetical order:

Alteplase
Atorvastatin
Amiodarone
Amlodipine
Aspirin
Atenolol
Atropine
Captopril
Clopidogrel
Digoxin
Diltiazem
Dobutamine
Dopamine
Enalapril
Enoxaparin
Epinephrine
Furosemide
Heparin
Hydralazine
Hydrochlorothiazide
Lisinopril
Losartan
Metoprolol
Nifedipine
Nitroprusside
Norepinephrine
Procainamide
Propranolol
Streptokinase
Vasopressin
Verapamil
Warfarin

AT A GLANCE

Use the color test page at the back of this book to see what your favorite colors look like on the page. Then, use this page to assign colors to medications grouped by therapeutic class.

Blood Thinners

Alteplase

Aspirin

Clopidogrel

Enoxaparin

Heparin

Streptokinase

Warfarin

Lipid Lowering Agent

Atorvastatin

Diuretic

Furosemide

Anti-Arrhythmics

Amiodarone

Atropine

Digoxin

Procainamide

Inotropics

Dobutamin

Dopamine

Vasopressors

Epinephrine

Norepinephrine

Vasopressin

Antihypertensives

Amlodipine

Captopril

Diltiazem

Elanapril

Hydralazine

Hydrochlorothiazide

Lisinopril

Losartan

Atenolol

Metoprolol

Nifedipine

Nitroprusside

Propranolol

Verapamil

DISCLAIMER

Therapeutic Class

THROMBOLYTIC

ALTEPLASE

Pharmacological Class

PLASMINOGEN ACTIVATOR

ALTEPLASE

Trade Name

tPA, Activase

Indication

MI, Ischemic Stroke, Occluded Central Lines

Action

Converts plasminogen to plasmin, degrades fibrin

Nursing Considerations

- Contraindicated if patient is actively bleeding
- Monitor closely for signs of bleeding (petechiae)
- May cause intracranial hemorrhage
- Use caution in setting of uncontrolled hypertension
- Assess neurological status frequently

Notes

_____
_____
_____
_____
_____
_____
_____
_____

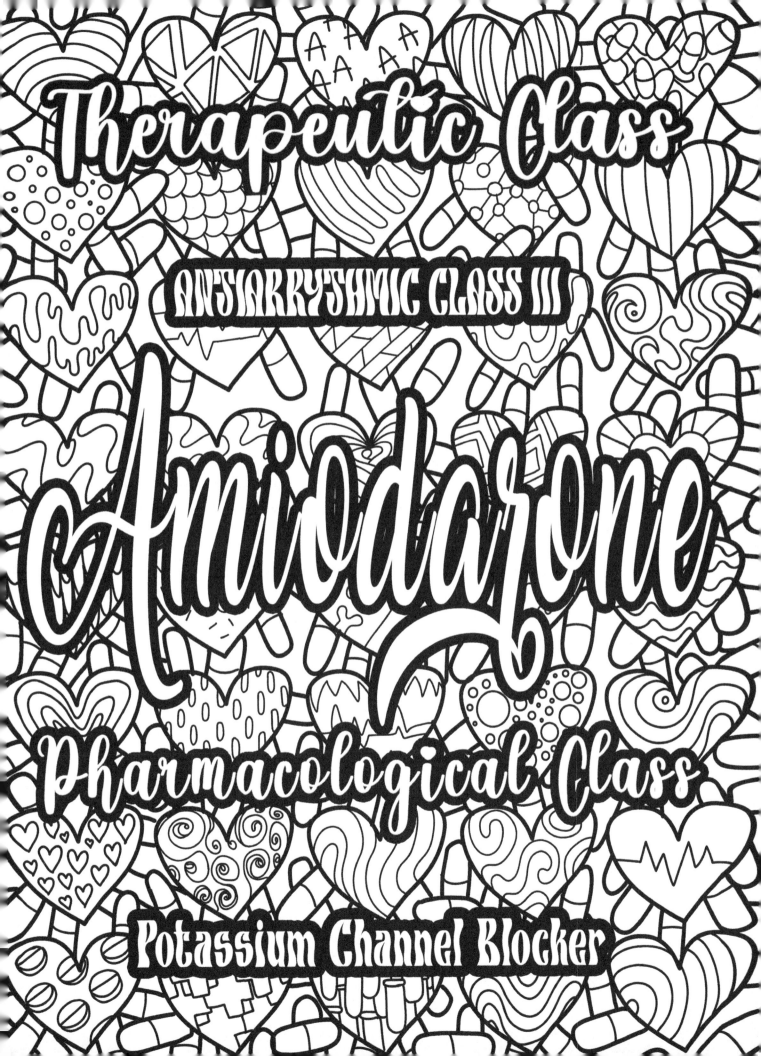

Therapeutic Class

ANTIARRYTHMIC CLASS III

Amiodarone

Pharmacological Class

Potassium Channel Blocker

AMIODARONE

Trade Name
Cordarone

Indication
A-FIB, Ventricular Dysrhythmias, SVT, ACLS Protocol for V-FIB and V-TACH

Action
Inhibits adrenergic stimulation, prolongs phase 3 of the action potential, thereby slowing the heart rate

Nursing Considerations
- Avoid grapefruit juice while on drug therapy
- Increases risk for QT prolongation
- Increases digoxin levels
- Increases activity of warfarin
- May lead to ARDS, CHF, bradycardia, and hypotension
- Monitor EKG continuously while on drug therapy
- Monitor liver function tests
- Teach patient to check pulse daily and report abnormalities

Notes
_____
_____
_____
_____
_____
_____

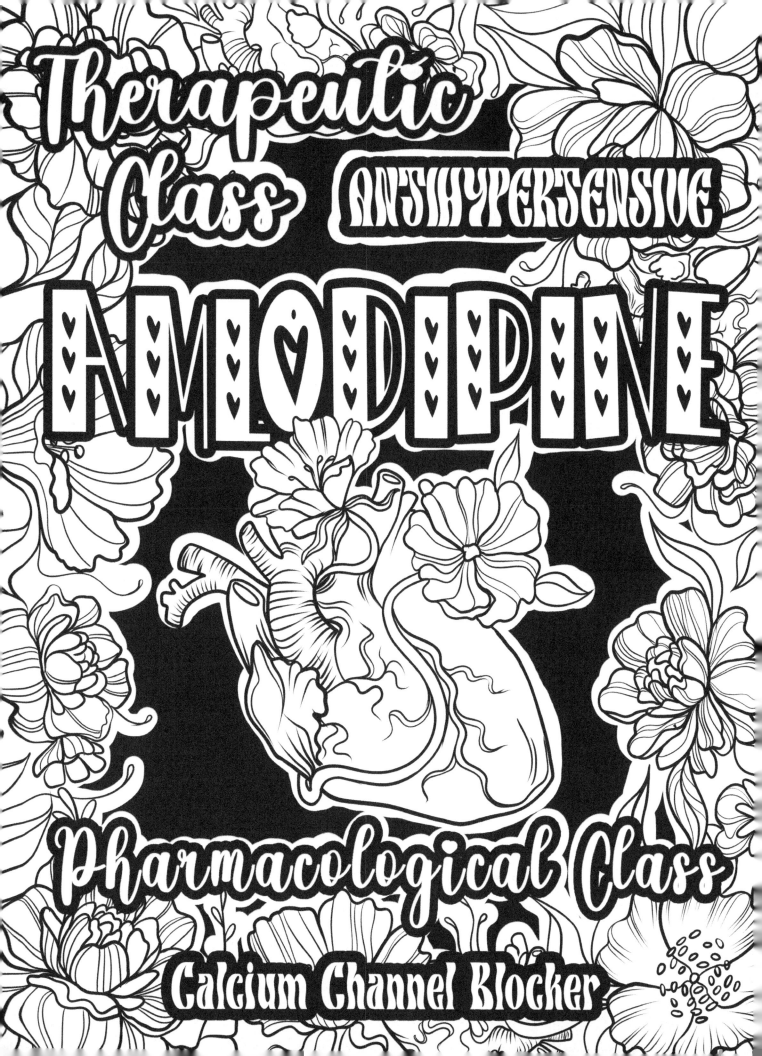

AMLODIPINE

Trade Name

Norvasc

Indication

Hypertension, Angina

Action

Blocks transport of calcium ions into muscle cells, inhibiting excitation and contraction

Nursing Considerations

- May cause gingival hyperplasia
- Grapefruit juice may increase drug levels
- Assess for signs of CHF
- Monitor blood pressure and heart rate prior to and during drug therapy
- Monitor intake and output
- Teach patient how to take blood pressure and report abnormalities

Notes

_____

_____

_____

_____

_____

_____

Therapeutic Class

ANTIPYRETIC / ANALGESIC

ASPIRIN

Pharmacological Class

SALICYLATE

ASPIRIN

Generic Name

Acetylsalicylic Acid / ASA

Indication

Stroke and MI Prophylaxis, Arthritis

Action

Inhibits the production of prostaglandins,
and decreases platelet aggregation

Nursing Considerations

- Use with caution in bleeding disorders, ETOH abuse
- May lead to Stevens-Johnson Syndrome
- Increased risk of bleeding with warfarin, heparin, and clopidogrel
- Increased risk of GI bleeding with NSAIDs, ETOH
- Monitor liver function tests
- Aspirin with viral infections may cause Reye's Syndrome

Notes

Therapeutic Class

ANTIANGINAL / ANTIHYPERTENSIVE

ATENOLOL

Pharmacological Class

BETA BLOCKER

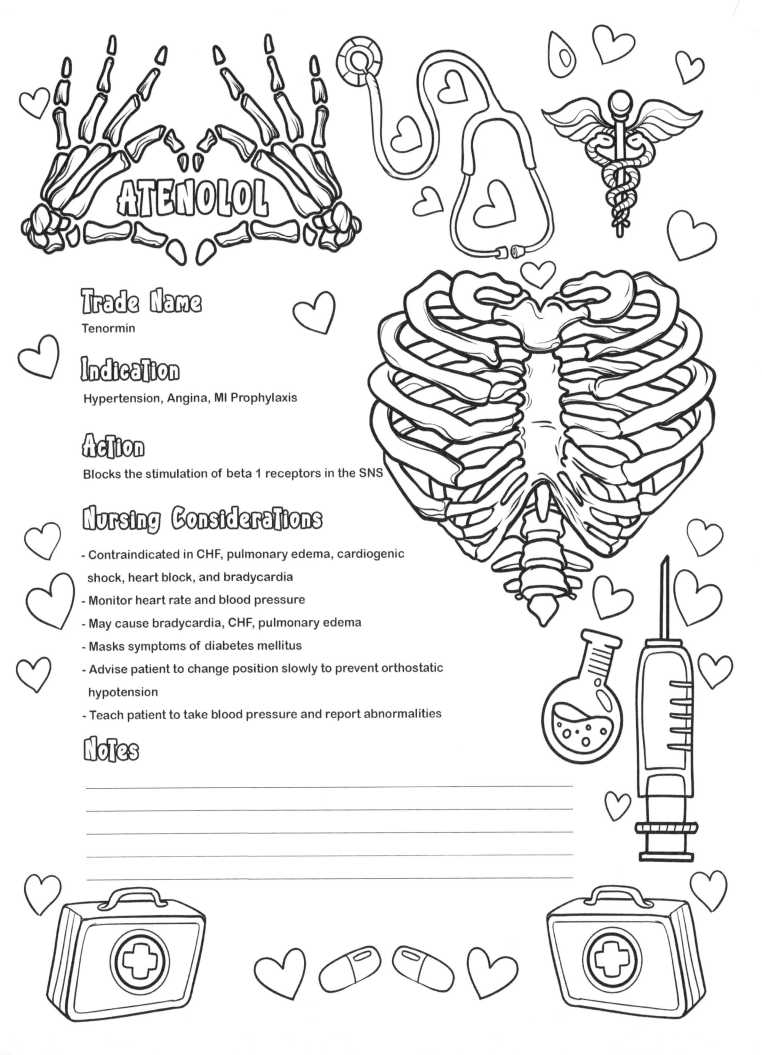

ATENOLOL

Trade Name
Tenormin

Indication
Hypertension, Angina, MI Prophylaxis

Action
Blocks the stimulation of beta 1 receptors in the SNS

Nursing Considerations

- Contraindicated in CHF, pulmonary edema, cardiogenic shock, heart block, and bradycardia
- Monitor heart rate and blood pressure
- May cause bradycardia, CHF, pulmonary edema
- Masks symptoms of diabetes mellitus
- Advise patient to change position slowly to prevent orthostatic hypotension
- Teach patient to take blood pressure and report abnormalities

Notes

_____
_____
_____
_____

Therapeutic Class
LIPID LOWERING AGENTS
ATORVASTATIN
Pharmacological Class
HMG-COA REDUCTASE INHIBITOR

ATORVASTATIN

Trade Name

Lipitor

Indication

Management of high cholesterol, primary prevention of cardiovascular disease

Action

Inhibits HMG-CoA Reductase in the liver, lowering total cholesterol as well as LDL

Nursing Considerations

- Contraindicated in liver disease
- Monitor liver function
- Monitor renal function
- May cause rhabdomyolysis
- Instruct patient to report muscle weakness (sign of rhabdomyolysis)
- Monitor serum cholesterol before starting, 4 weeks post initiation, and frequently throughout drug therapy

Notes

Therapeutic Class

ANTIARRHYSHMIC

ATROPINE

Pharmacological Class

ANTICHOLINERGIC / ANTIMUSCARINIC

ATROPINE

Trade Name
Atro-Pen

Indication
Symptomatic Bradycardia, Heart Block, Bronchospasm, Excessive Secretions

Action
Inhibits the parasympathetic nervous system, specifically acetylcholine

Nursing Considerations
- Avoid use in hemorrhage, tachycardia, and close angle glaucoma
- Monitor for tachycardia and palpitations
- May cause urinary retention
- May cause constipation

Notes
_____
_____
_____
_____
_____
_____
_____
_____

ANTIHYPERTENSIVE

Captopril

ACE INHIBITOR

CAPTOPRIL

Trade Name

Capoten

Indication

Hypertension, CHF, DM Neuropathy

Action

Blocks conversion of angiotensin I to angiotensin II, increases renin and decreases aldosterone

Nursing Considerations

- May cause rhabdomyolysis

- Can cause neutropenia - check WBC's

- Use with caution with potassium supplements

- Use with caution with diuretics

- Monitor blood pressure, weight, and fluid status

- Administer 1 hour before meals

- Most common side effect: dry cough

Notes

Therapeutic Class

ANTIPLATELET

CLOPIDOGREL

Pharmacological Class

PLATELET INHIBITOR

CLOPIDOGREL

Trade Name

Plavix

Indication

MI / ACS, CVA, PVD, and Atherosclerotic Disease

Action

Inhibits platelet aggregation

Nursing Considerations

- May cause GI bleeding, neutropenia, hypercholesterolemia
- Increased risk of bleeding with warfarin, aspirin, heparin
- Increased risk of bleeding with garlic, ginkgo, ginger
- Monitor of signs and symptoms of bleeding
- Monitor CBC and Platelet Count
- Discontinue 5 - 7 days before surgery

Notes

_____

_____

_____

_____

_____

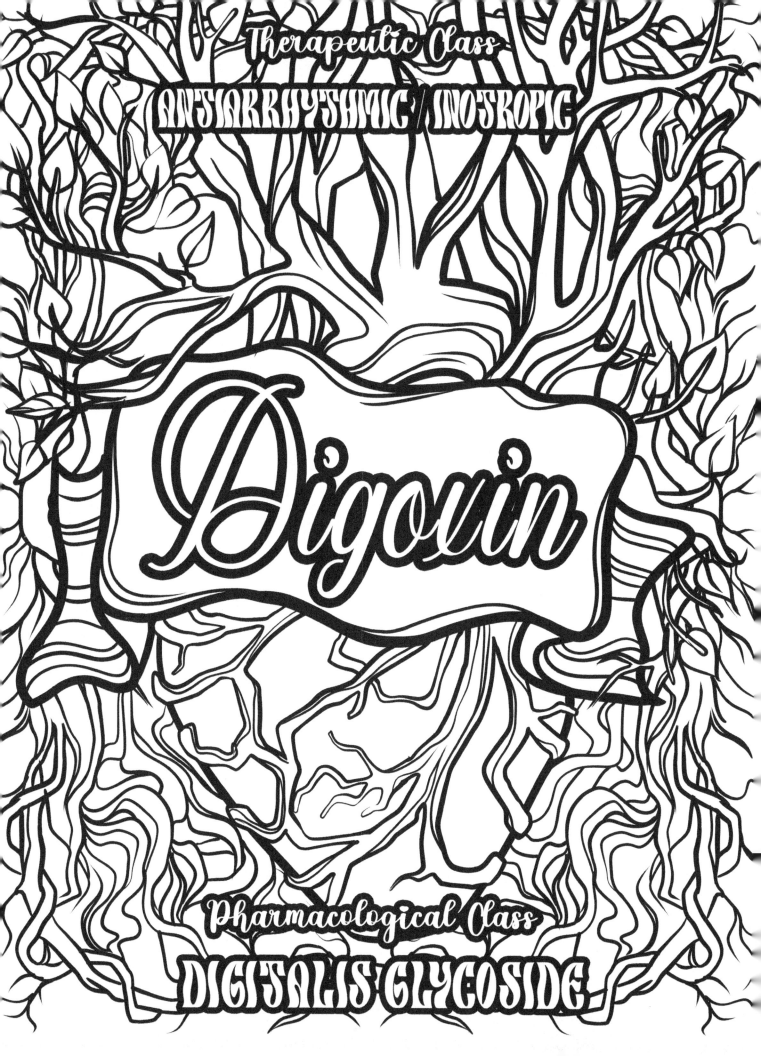

DIGOXIN

Trade Name

Lanoxin

Indication

CHF, A-FIB, A-Flutter

Action

Increases myocardial contractility, prolongs the refractory period, and decreases conduction through the SA and AV nodes, thereby increasing cardiac output while simultaneously slowing the heart rate.

Nursing Considerations

- Contraindicated in uncontrolled ventricular dysrhythmias
- Excreted by the kidneys
- Hypokalemia increases risk for toxicity
- Hypercalcemia increases risk for toxicity
- Use with caution with diuretics
- Assess for bradycardia - Monitor heart rate for 1 full minute prior to administration
- Signs of toxicity include blurred vision and yellow/green visual disturbances

Notes

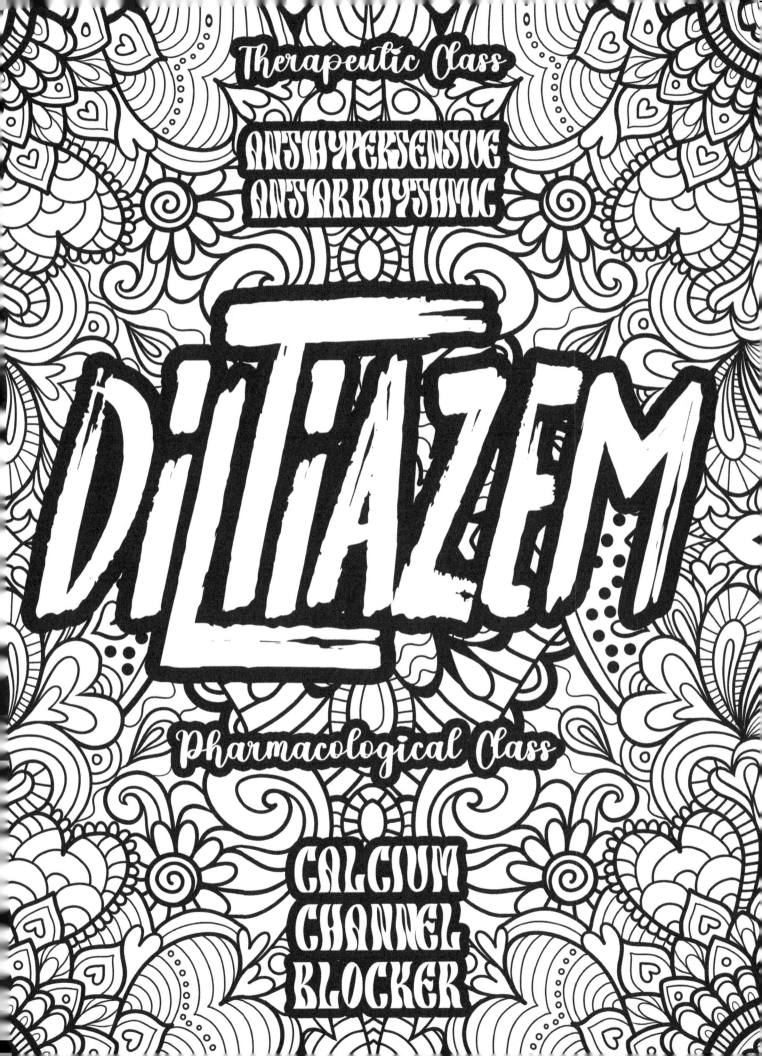

Therapeutic Class

ANTIHYPERTENSIVE
ANTIARRHYTHMIC

DILTIAZEM

Pharmacological Class

CALCIUM
CHANNEL
BLOCKER

DILTIAZEM

Trade Name

Cardizem

Indication

Hypertension, SVT, A-FIB, A-Flutter, Angina

Action

Inhibits calcium transport resulting in decreased excitation and contraction, depressing the SA and NA nodes and increasing vasodilation

Nursing Considerations

- Contraindicated in 2nd and 3rd degree AV Block
- May cause CHF, bradycardia, and gingival hyperplasia
- Increases digoxin levels
- Instruct patient to not drink grapefruit juice
- Assess for signs and symptoms of CHF
- Monitor EKG continuously
- Monitor serum potassium
- Teach patient how to take blood pressure and report abnormalities

Notes

_____
_____
_____
_____
_____

Therapeutic Class

INOTROPIC

DOBUTAMINE

Pharmacological Class

BETA ADRENERGIC AGONIST

DOBUTAMINE

Trade Name

Dubotrex

Indication

Short term management of heart failure

Action

Stimulates Beta 1 receptors in the heart, producing an inotropic effect that increases cardiac output with little effect on heart rate.

Nursing Considerations

- Monitor hemodynamics: blood pressure, heart rate, and ectopy
- Monitor peripheral pulses
- Skin reactions may occur with hypersensitivity
- Instruct patient to not drink grapefruit juice
- Beta Blockers may negate effects

Notes

_____
_____
_____
_____
_____
_____
_____

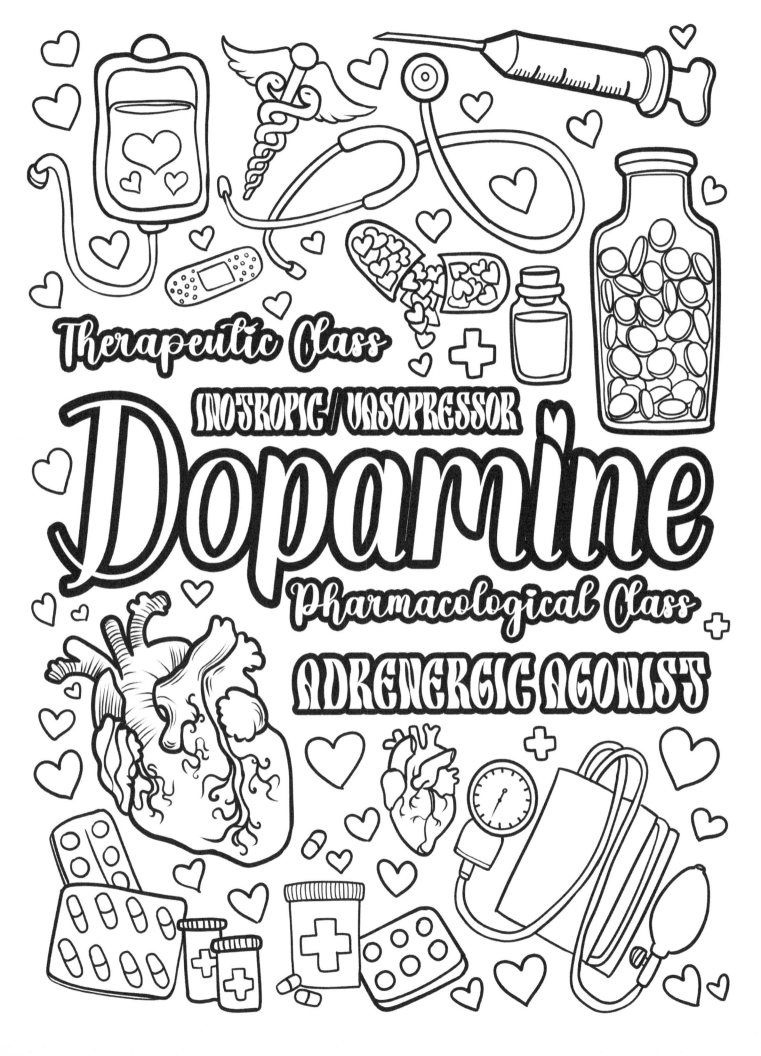

Therapeutic Class

INOTROPIC/VASOPRESSOR

Dopamine

Pharmacological Class

ADRENERGIC AGONIST

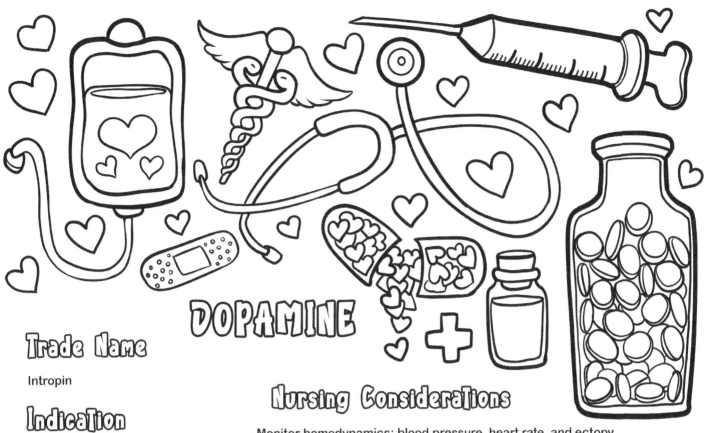

DOPAMINE

Trade Name

Intropin

Indication

Short term management of shock.
Improves cardiac output,
blood pressure, and urine output.

Action

Small doses produce renal vasodilation.
Doses 2 - 10 mcg/kg/min produce beta
1 stimulation, increasing cardiac output.
Doses >10 mcg/kg/min produce
alpha stimulation, increasing vasoconstriction.

Nursing Considerations

- Monitor hemodynamics: blood pressure, heart rate, and ectopy
- Monitor peripheral pulses
- Titrate to obtain blood pressure goal
- Assess for irritation at IV site
- Beta blockers may negate effects

Notes

_____
_____
_____
_____
_____

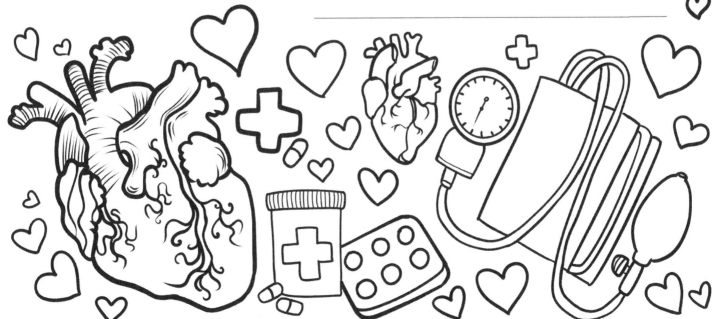

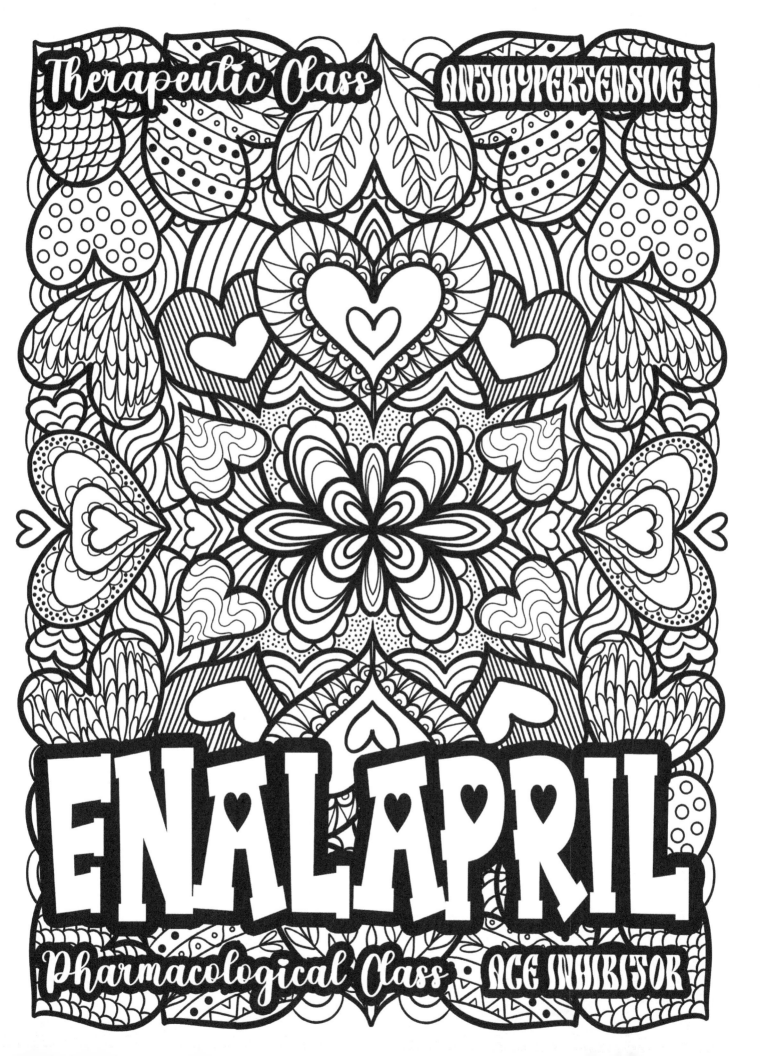

Therapeutic Class   ANTIHYPERTENSIVE

ENALAPRIL

Pharmacological Class   ACE INHIBITOR

ENALAPRIL

Trade Name

Vasotec

Indication

Hypertension, CHF

Action

Blocks conversion for angiotensin I to angiotensin II, increasing renin levels and decreasing aldosterone, leading to vasodilation

Nursing Considerations

- Can cause neutropenia – Monitor WBC's
- Caution with potassium supplements
- Caution with diuretics
- Monitor blood pressure, weight, and fluid status
- Monitor renal panel
- Administer 1 hour before meals
- Common side effect: dry cough

Notes

_____
_____
_____
_____
_____

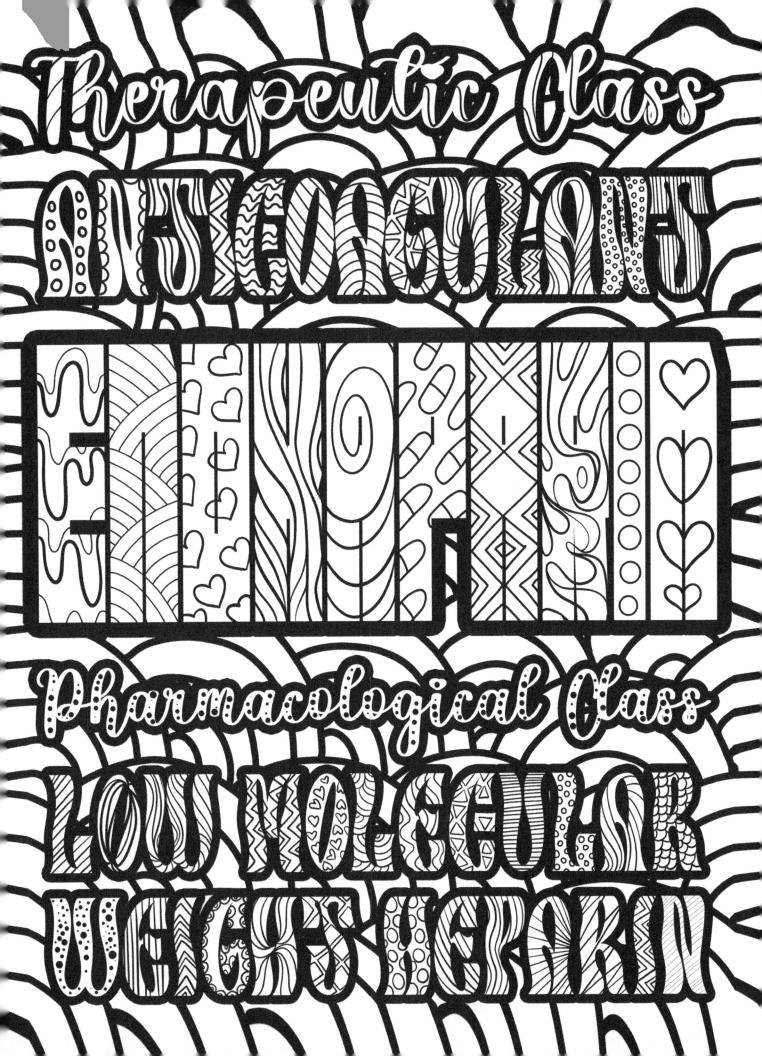

Therapeutic Class

ANTICOAGULANTS

HEPARIN

Pharmacological Class

LOW MOLECULAR WEIGHT HEPARIN

Trade Name

Lovenox

Indication

Prevention of DVT, PE, and VTE

Action

Potentiates the inhibitory effect of antithrombin on factor Xa and thrombin, preventing thrombus formation.

Nursing Considerations

- Contraindicated in pork hypersensitivity
- Monitor for signs of bleeding
- Administer in subcutaneous tissue
- DO NOT eject air bubble prior to administration
- DO NOT aspirate or massage site

Notes

ENOXAPARIN

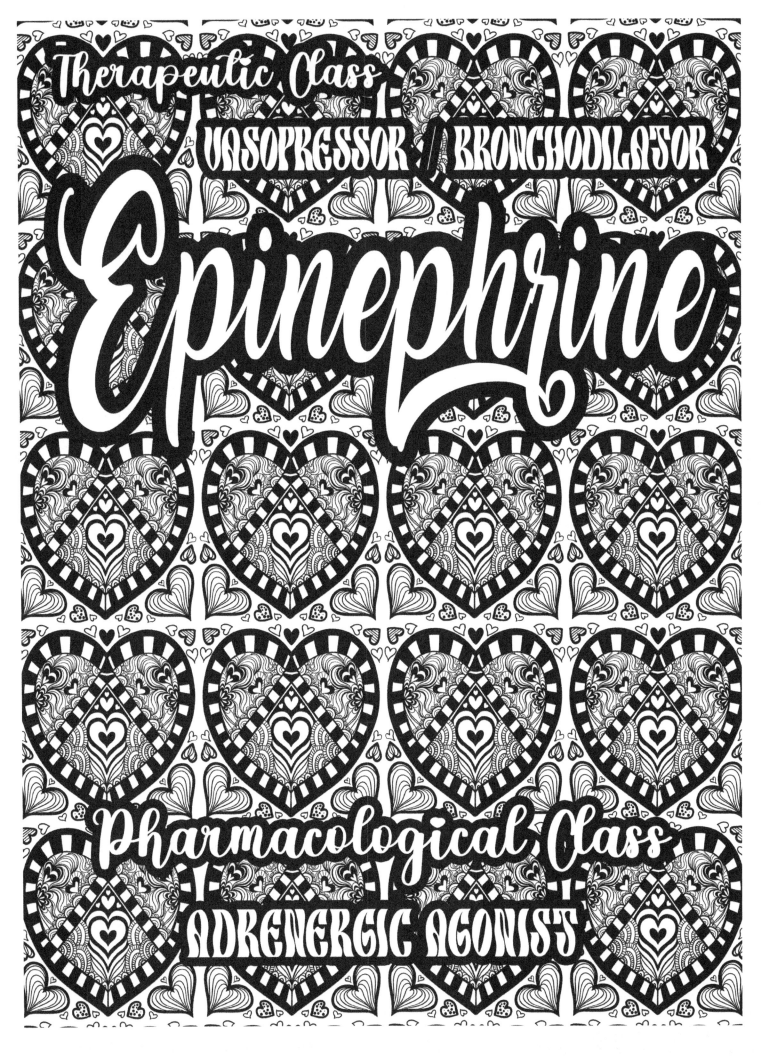

Therapeutic Class

VASOPRESSOR / BRONCHODILATOR

Epinephrine

Pharmacological Class

ADRENERGIC AGONIST

EPINEPHRINE

Trade Name

Adrenalin, EpiPen

Indication

Cardiac Arrest, Allergic Reactions, Asthma and COPD Exacerbations

Action

Stimulates Beta 1, Beta 2, and Alpha receptors, resulting in bronchodilation, increased heart rate, and increased blood pressure.

Nursing Considerations

- Side eects: angina, tachycardia, hypertension, restlessness,
 and hyperglycemia
- Use with MAOI's may precipitate a hypertensive crises
- Monitor for chest pain
- Assess lung sounds, heart rate and blood pressure
- Rinse mouth after inhalation
- Beta Blockers may negate effects

Notes

_____
_____
_____
_____
_____
_____
_____

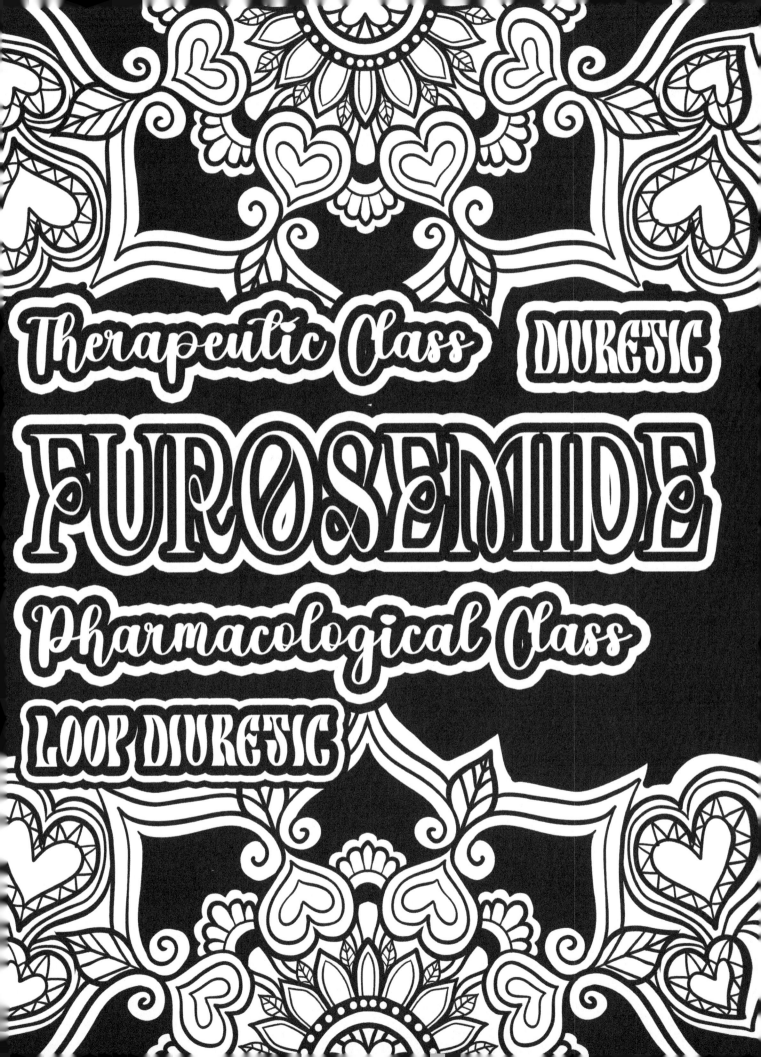

Therapeutic Class DIURETIC

FUROSEMIDE

Pharmacological Class

LOOP DIURETIC

FUROSEMIDE

Trade Name

Lasix

Indication

Hypertension, Edema

Action

Prevents reabsorption of sodium and chloride in the kidneys, increasing excretion of water, sodium, chloride, magnesium, and potassium.

Nursing Considerations

- Caution with liver disease
- May cause hypotension, dehydration, electrolyte imbalance, and metabolic alkalosis
- Hypokalemia may lead to increased risk for digoxin toxicity
- Monitor renal panel
- Do not administer with aminoglycosides due to ototoxicity

Notes

_____
_____
_____
_____
_____

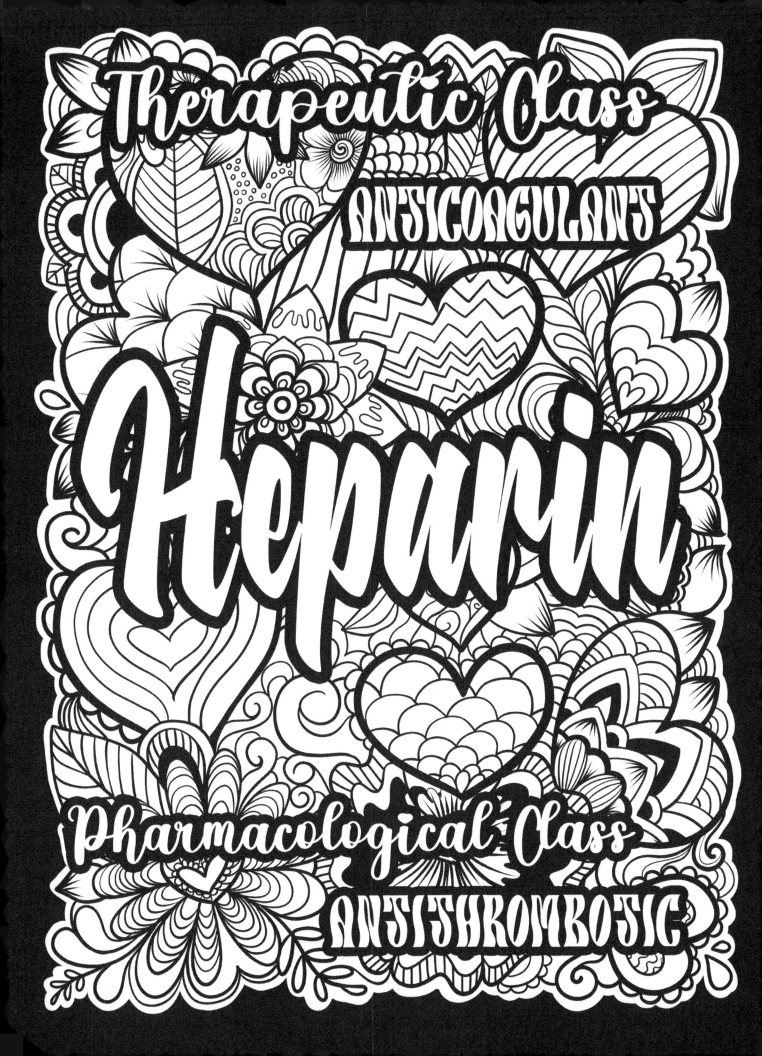

HEPARIN

Trade Name

Hep-Lock

Indication

Venous Thromboembolism, IV Catheter Clotting

Action

Potentiates the inhibitory effect of antithrombin on factor Xa and thrombin, preventing thrombus formation.

Nursing Considerations

- Monitor for signs and symptoms of bleeding
- Monitor platelet count
- May cause hyperkalemia
- Teach patient to report any signs of bleeding

Notes

_____
_____
_____
_____
_____
_____

Therapeutic Class

ANTIHYPERTENSIVE

HYDRALAZINE

Pharmacological Class

VASODILATOR

HYDRALAZINE

Trade Name

Apresoline

Indication

Hypertension

Action

Causes arterial vasodilation, exact mechanism unknown.

Nursing Considerations

- May cause tachycardia, sodium retention, and angina

- Monitor blood pressure

- Caution with MAOI's

- Teach patient how to take blood pressure and report abnormalities

Notes

_____

_____

_____

_____

_____

_____

_____

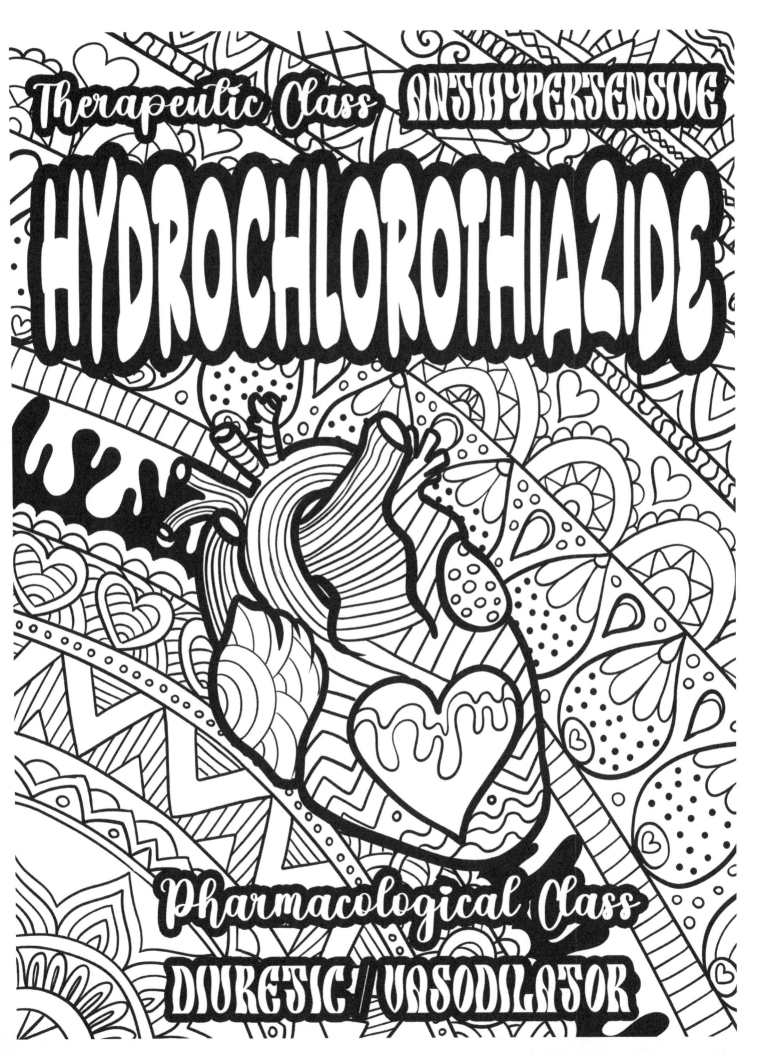

Therapeutic Class ANTIHYPERTENSIVE

HYDROCHLOROTHIAZIDE

Pharmacological Class

DIURETIC / VASODILATOR

HYDROCHLOROTHIAZIDE

Trade Name

HydroDiuril

Indication

Hypertension, CHF, Renal Dysfunction, Cirrhosis, Glucocorticoid Therapy

Action

Increases sodium and water excretion and produces arterial vasodilation

Nursing Considerations

- May cause dizziness, hypokalemia, hyponatremia, hypophosphatemia, hypomagnesemia, and dehydration
- Hypokalemia can increase risk for digoxin toxicity
- Monitor blood pressure and I's & O's
- Monitor electrolytes
- Administer at the same time each day, even if symptoms improve
- Teach patient how to take blood pressure and report abnormalities

Notes

_____
_____
_____
_____
_____

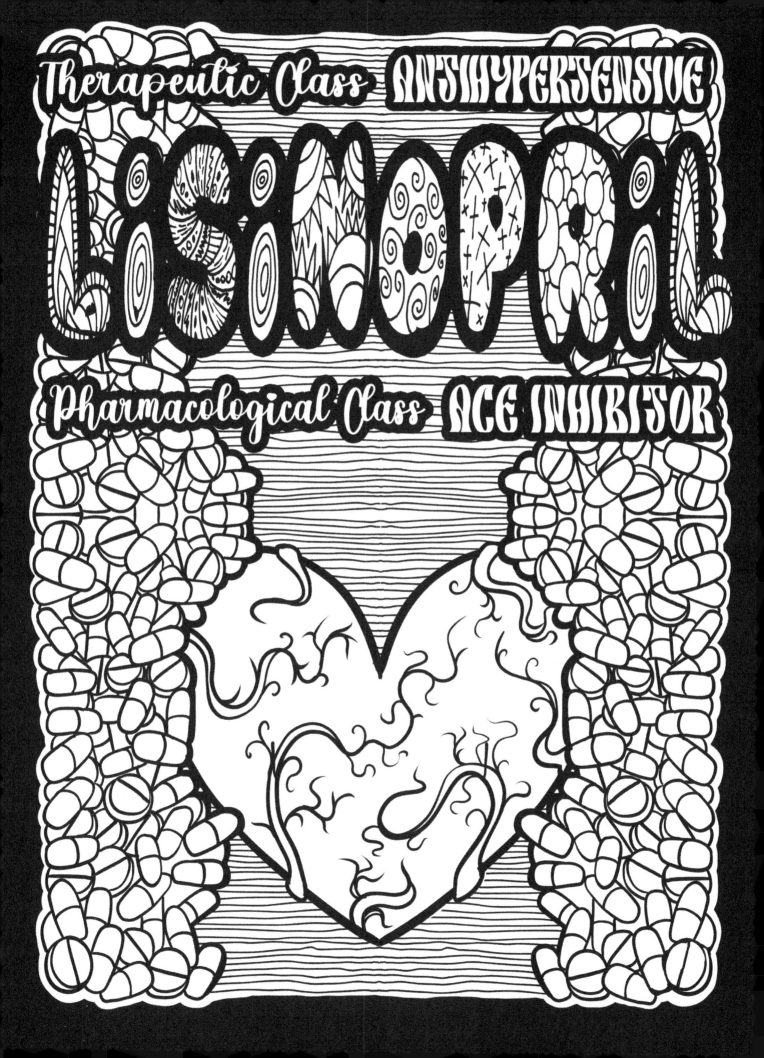

LISINOPRIL

Trade Name
Prinivil

Indication
Hypertension, CHF

Action
Blocks conversion of angiotensin I to angiotensin II, increasing renin and decreasing aldosterone leading to vasodilation.

Nursing Considerations
- Common side effect: dry cough
- Caution: first does may cause profound hypotension
- Caution with potassium supplements and potassium sparing diuretics
- Caution with diuretic therapy
- Monitor blood pressure
- Monitor weight and fluid status
- Monitor renal and liver function tests
- Administer 1 hour before meals

Notes

_____
_____
_____
_____
_____
_____
_____
_____

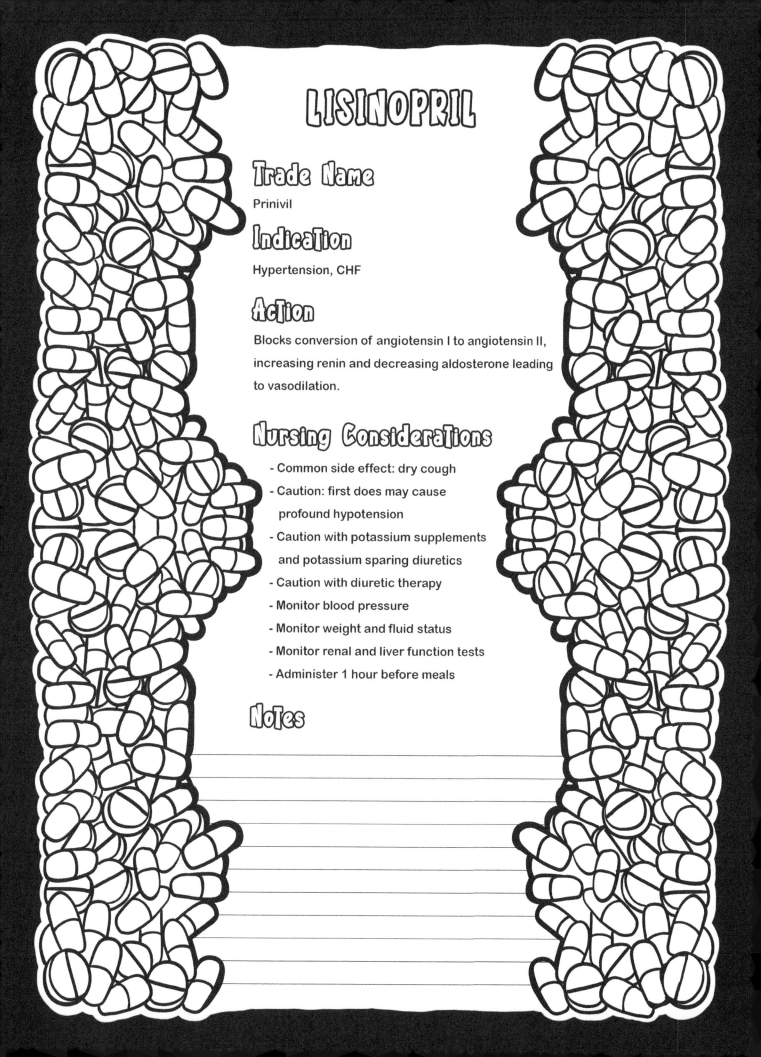

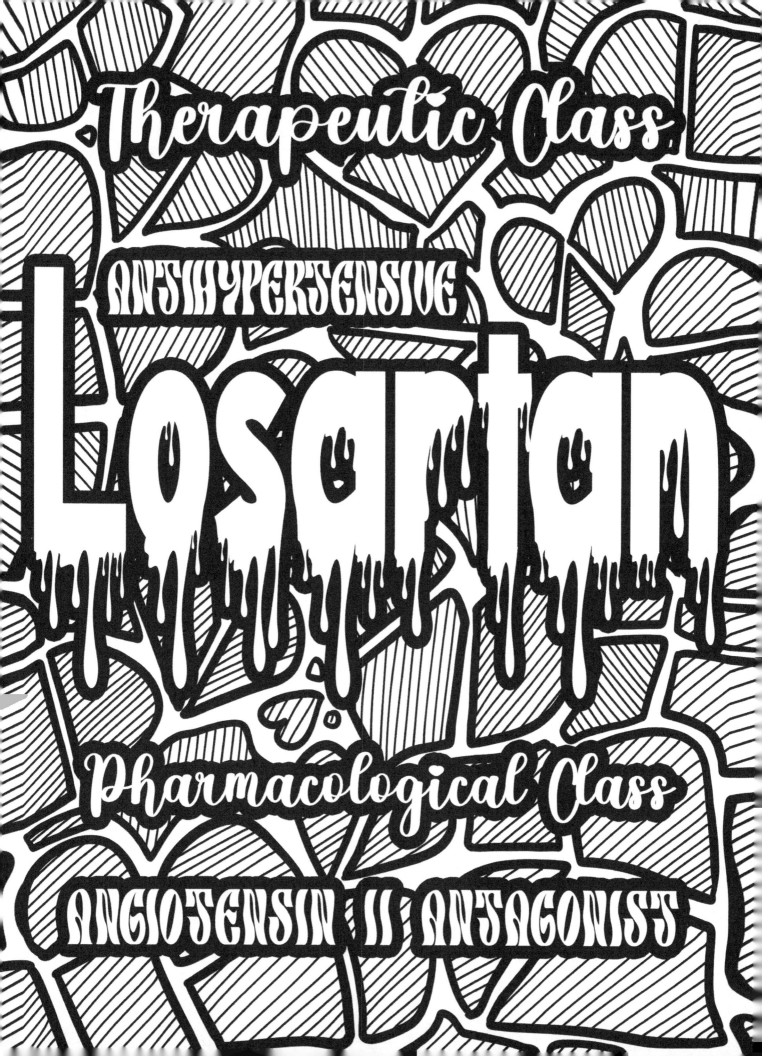

Therapeutic Class

ANTIHYPERTENSIVE

Losartan

Pharmacological Class

ANGIOTENSIN II ANTAGONIST

LOSARTAN

Trade Name

Cozaar

Indication

Hypertension, CHF, Diabetic Neuropathy

Action

Inhibits the vasoconstrictive properties of angiotensin II.

Nursing Considerations

- May cause hypotension, tachycardia, angioedema, hyperkalemia
- May increase digoxin levels
- Assess blood pressure and heart rate
- Assess fluid status
- Monitor daily weights
- Monitor renal and liver function tests
- Teach patient to take blood pressure and report abnormalities

Notes

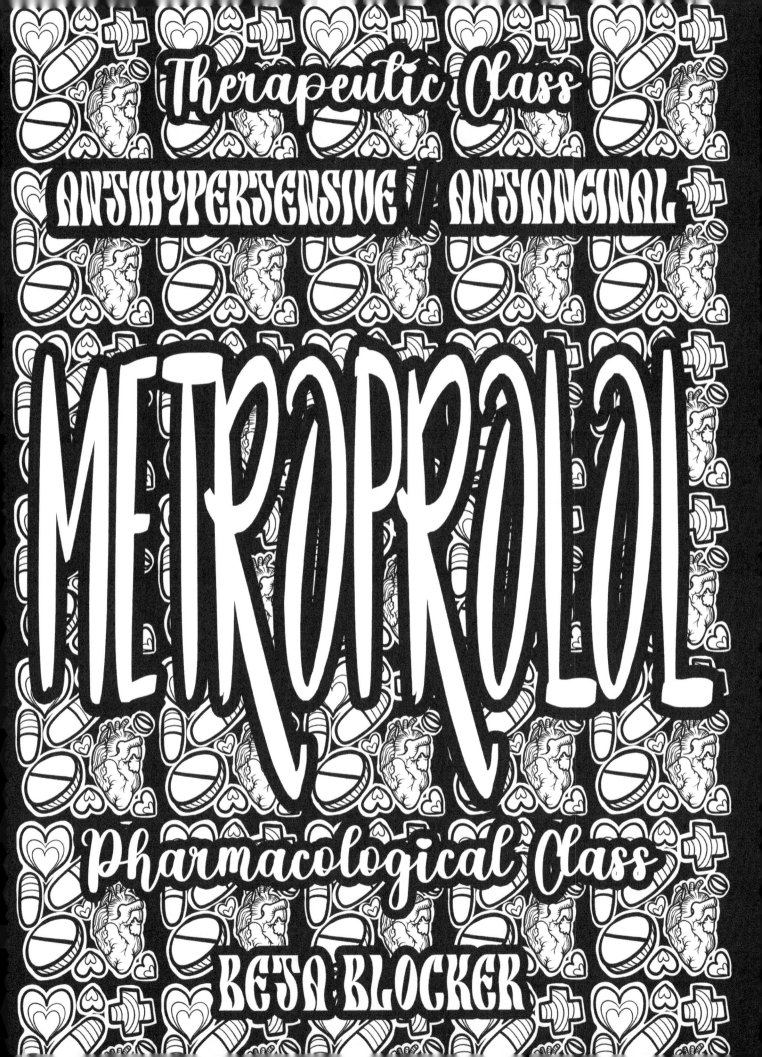

Therapeutic Class

ANTIHYPERTENSIVE / ANTIANGINAL

METOPROLOL

Pharmacological Class

BETA BLOCKER

METROPROLOL

Trade Name

Lopressor

Indication

Hypertension, Angina, Tachyarrhythmias, CHF, Migraine Prophylaxis

Action

Blocks the stimulation of Beta 1 receptors.

Nursing Considerations

- Monitor hemodynamics
- May lead to bradycardia, pulmonary edema
- Caution with MAOI's
- Monitor for signs and symptoms of CHF

Notes

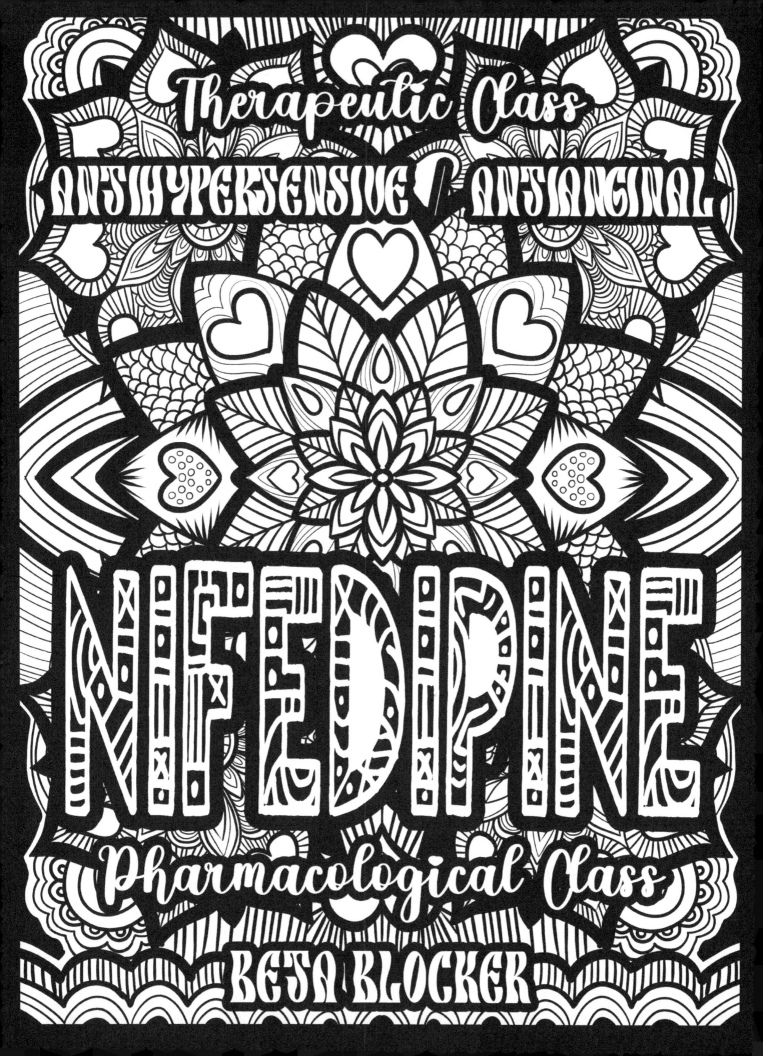

Therapeutic Class

ANTIHYPERTENSIVE ANTIANGINAL

NIFEDIPINE

Pharmacological Class

BETA BLOCKER

NIFEDIPINE

Trade Name

Procardia

Indication

Hypertension, Angina, CHF, Migraine Prophylaxis

Action

Blocks calcium transport resulting in inhibition of contraction, leading to vasodilation.

Nursing Considerations

- Teach patient to NOT consume grapefruit juice
- Caution in heart block, low blood pressure
- May cause dysrhythmias
- May cause gingival hyperplasia, Steven's Johnson Syndrome
- Monitor blood pressure and heart rate
- Teach patient to take blood pressure and report abnormalities

Notes

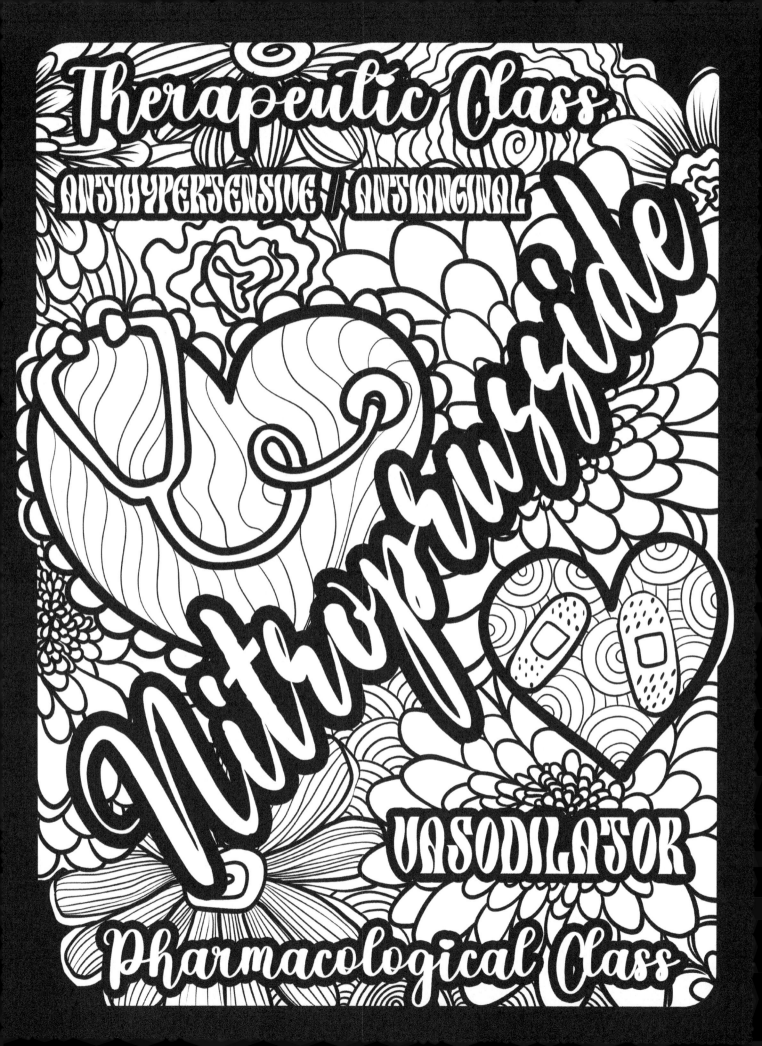

Therapeutic Class

ANTIHYPERTENSIVE / ANTIANGINAL

Nitroprusside

VASODILATOR

Pharmacological Class

NITROPRUSSIDE

Trade Name

Nitropress

Indication

Hypertensive Crisis, Cardiogenic Shock

Action

Converts to nitric oxide in the body, leading to smooth muscle relaxation and subsequent vasodilation.

Nursing Considerations

- Monitor heart rate, blood pressure, and EKG continuously
- May cause cyanide toxicity
- Sympathomimetics may decrease effectiveness

Notes

_____
_____
_____
_____
_____

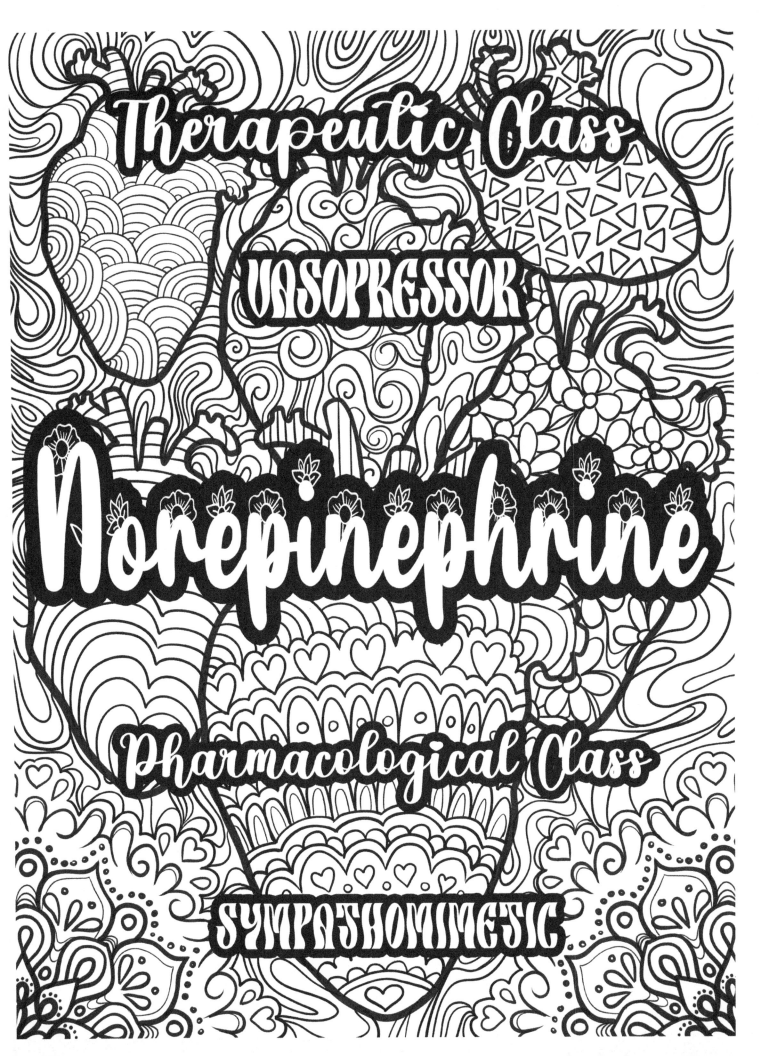

NOREPINEPHRINE

Trade Name

Levophed

Indication

Severe Hypotension, Shock

Action

Stimulates alpha receptors in blood vessels, causing vasoconstriction and increasing blood pressure.

Nursing Considerations

- Monitor heart rate, blood pressure, and EKG continuously
- May result in rebound hypotension when discontinued
- Double check all concentrations with second nurse
- Teach patient to report headaches, dizziness, or chest pain

Notes

_____
_____
_____
_____
_____
_____
_____
_____

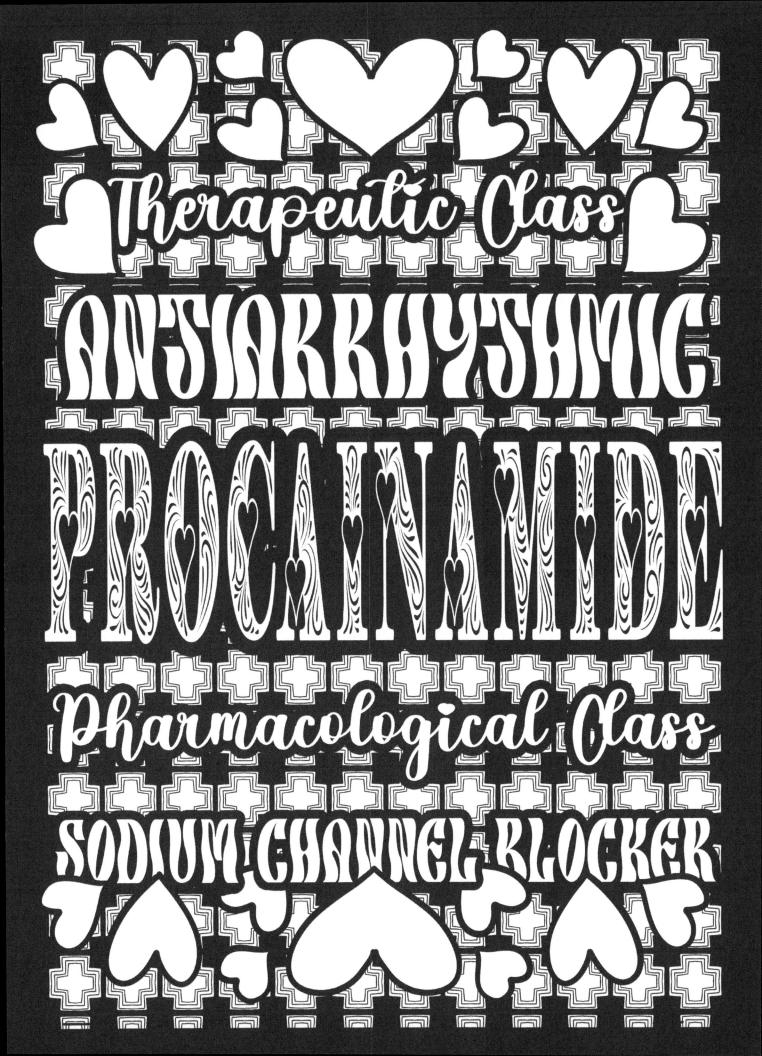

Therapeutic Class

ANTIARRHYTHMIC

PROCAINAMIDE

Pharmacological Class

SODIUM CHANNEL BLOCKER

PROCAINAMIDE

Trade Name

Procan

Indication

A wide variety of atrial and ventricular dysrhythmias, including V-TACH

Action

Inhibits sodium channels, slowing conduction and decreasing excitability throughout the heart.

Nursing Considerations

- May cause seizure, asystole, and heart block
- Monitor EKG continuously
- May cause hypotension; Keep patient supine
- Can cause drug induced lupus syndrome

Notes

_____
_____
_____
_____
_____
_____

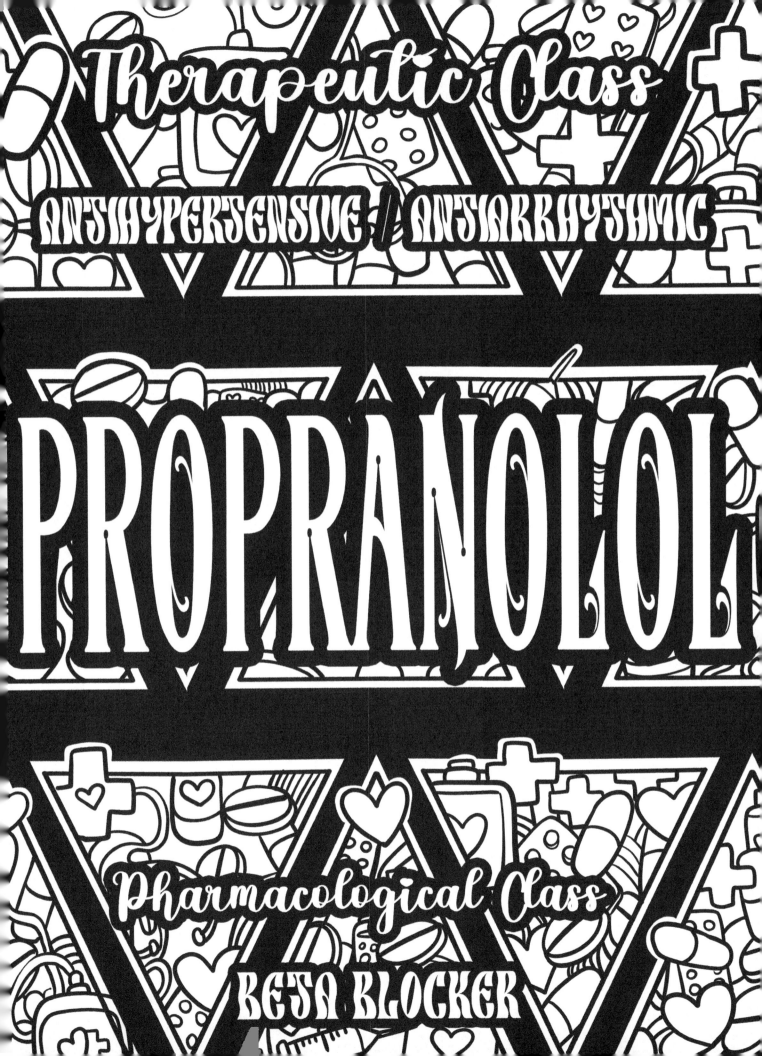

Therapeutic Class

ANTIHYPERTENSIVE / ANTIARRHYTHMIC

PROPRANOLOL

Pharmacological Class

BETA BLOCKER

PROPRANOLOL

Trade Name

Inderal

Indication

Hypertension, Arrhythmia, Angina, Alcohol Withdrawal

Action

Blocks Beta 1 and Beta 2 adrenergic receptors.

Nursing Considerations

- Contraindicated in CHF, cardiogenic shock, bradycardia, and heart block
- Monitor heart rate and blood pressure
- May cause bradycardia, CHF
- Masks symptoms of DM
- Teach patient to change position slowly to avoid orthostatic hypotension
- Stopping abruptly may result in life threatening arrhythmias

Notes

STREPTOKINASE

Therapeutic Class

THROMBOLYTIC

Pharmacological Class

PLASMINOGEN ACTIVATOR

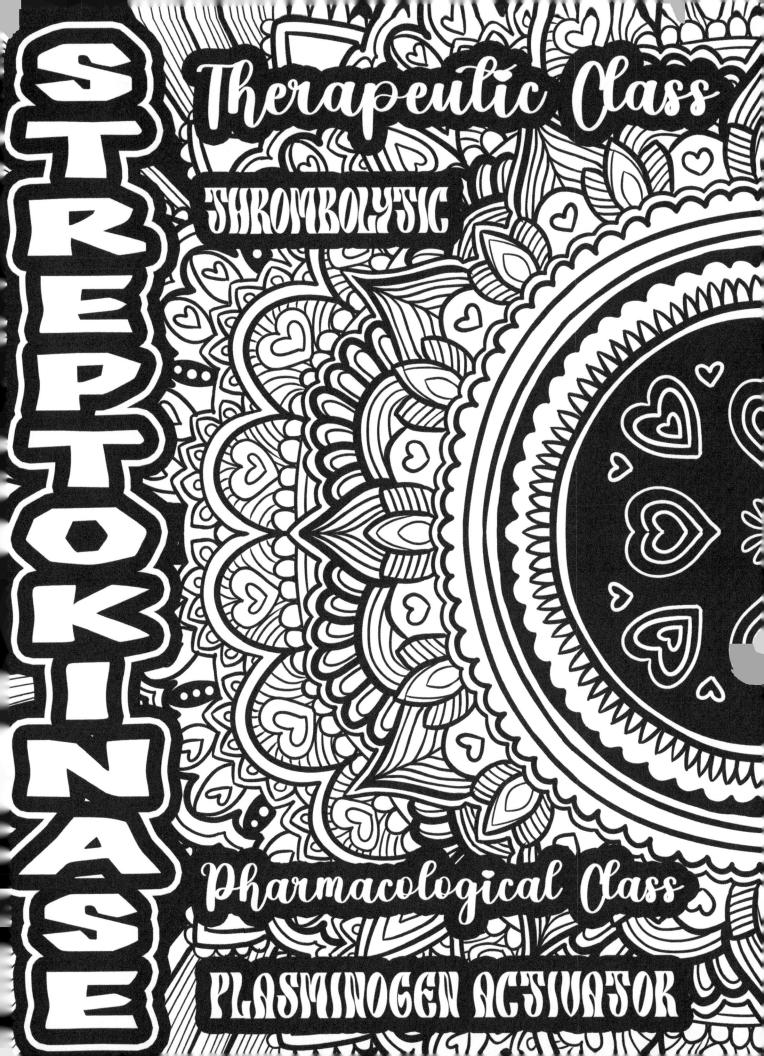

STREPTOKINASE

Trade Name

Streptase

Indication

PE, DVT, Occluded Lines

Action

Converts plasminogen to plasmin which degrades blood clots.

Nursing Considerations

- Contraindicated in active bleeding, bronchospasm, hypotension
- Monitor vital signs continuously
- Monitor for signs and symptoms of bleeding
- Avoid invasive procedures

Notes

_____

_____

_____

_____

_____

_____

_____

_____

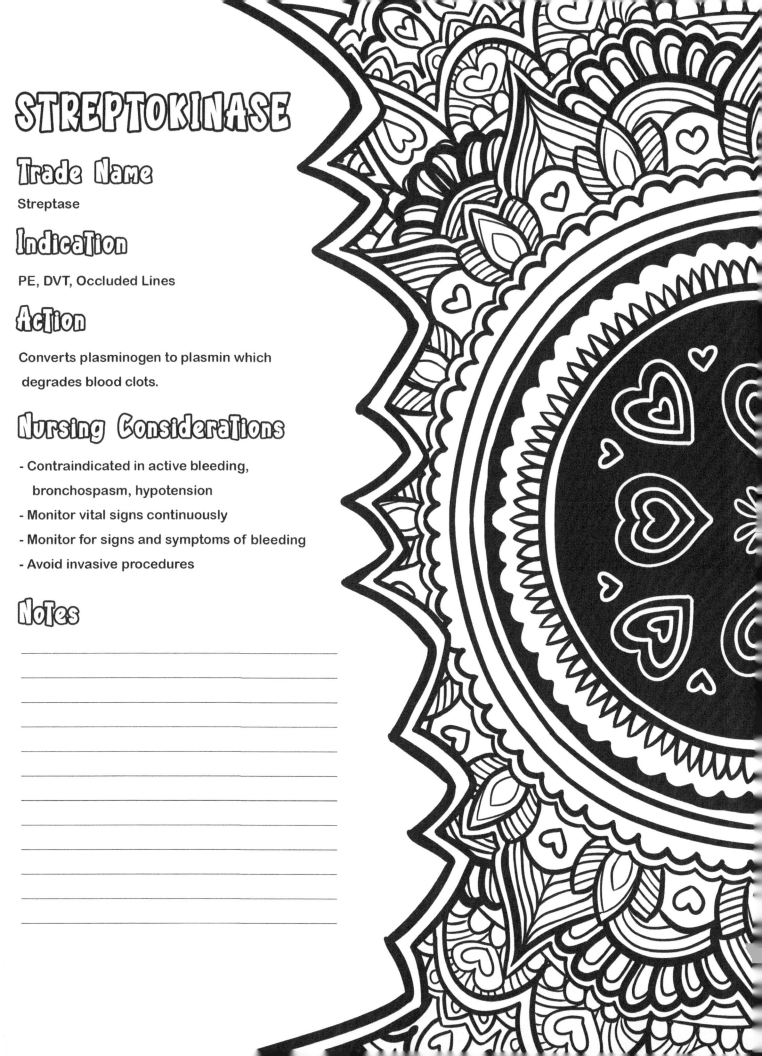

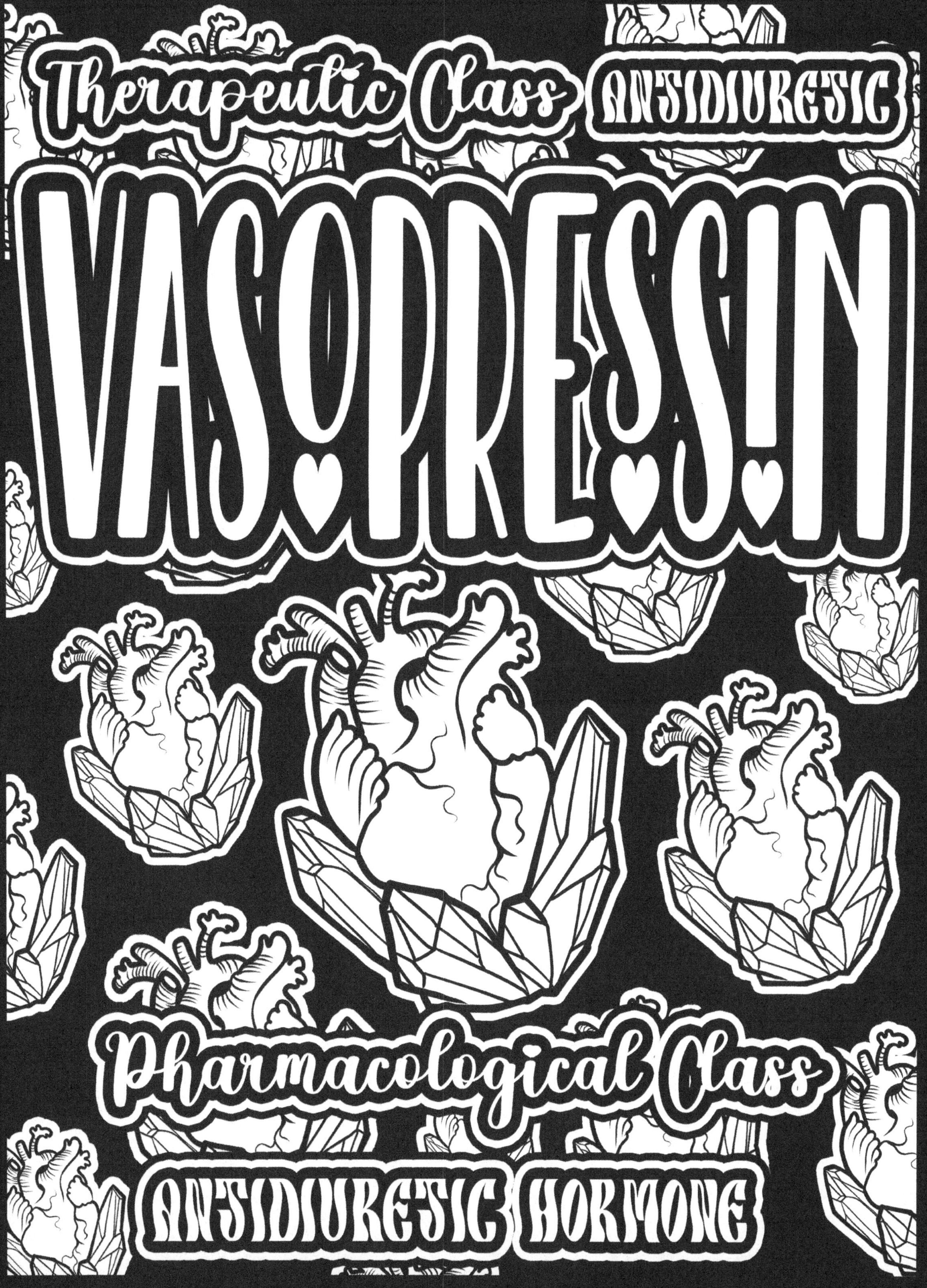

Therapeutic Class ANTIDIURETIC

VASOPRESSIN

Pharmacological Class

ANTIDIURETIC HORMONE

VASOPRESSIN

Trade Name

Pitressin

Indication

V-FIB / V-TACH unresponsive to initial shock, GI Hemorrhage,
Diabetes Insipidus

Action

Increases water permeability of the collecting duct and distal convoluted tubule
in the kidney, leading to water retention. Increases peripheral vascular
resistance leading to increased blood pressure.

Nursing Considerations

- Contraindicated in renal failure and hypersensitivity to pork
- Caution with heart failure and cardiovascular disease
- Monitor blood pressure, heart rate, and EKG
- Monitor urine specific gravity
- Perform daily weights
- Assess for edema

Notes

Therapeutic Class

ANTIHYPERTENSIVE
ANTIARRHYTHMIC

Verapamil

Pharmacological Class

CALCIUM CHANNEL BLOCKER

VERAPAMIL

Trade Name

Isoptin

Indication

Hypertension, Angina, SVT, Migraine

Action

Prevents transport of calcium, leading to decreased contraction.

Decreases conduction through SA and AV nodes.

Nursing Considerations

- Contraindicated in 2nd and 3rd degree heart block, hypotension

- May cause anxiety, confusion, CHF, bradycardia, hypotension

- Potentiated by grapefruit juice

- Can increase digoxin levels

- Monitor heart rate, blood pressure, and I's & O's

Notes

_____

_____

_____

_____

_____

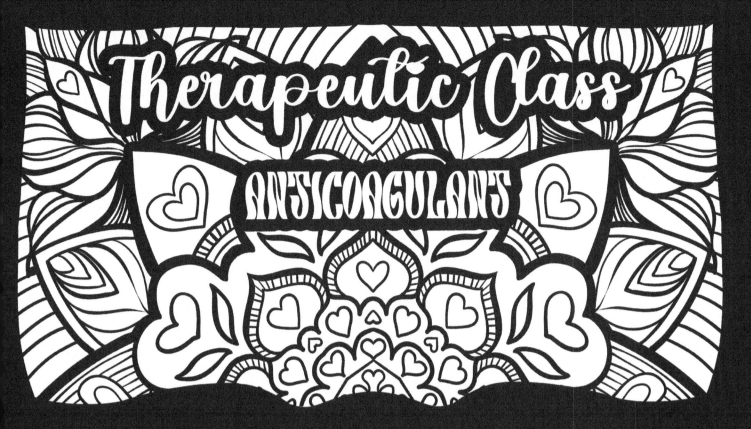

Therapeutic Class

ANTICOAGULANTS

WARFARIN

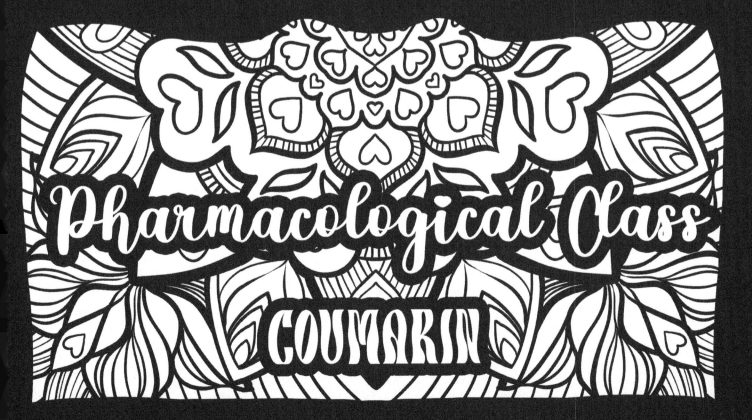

Pharmacological Class

COUMARIN

WARFARIN

Trade Name

Coumadin

Indication

Venous Thrombus, PE, A-FIB, MI

Action

Disrupts liver synthesis of Vitamin K dependent clotting factors.

Nursing Considerations

- Contraindicated in active bleeding, uncontrolled hypertension

- Can cause bleeding

- Azole antifungals, cimetidine increase effects

- Assess for signs and symptoms of bleeding

- Antidote is Vitamin K

- Teach patient to report signs and symptoms of bleeding

Notes

_____

_____

_____

_____

_____

_____

COLOR TEST PAGE

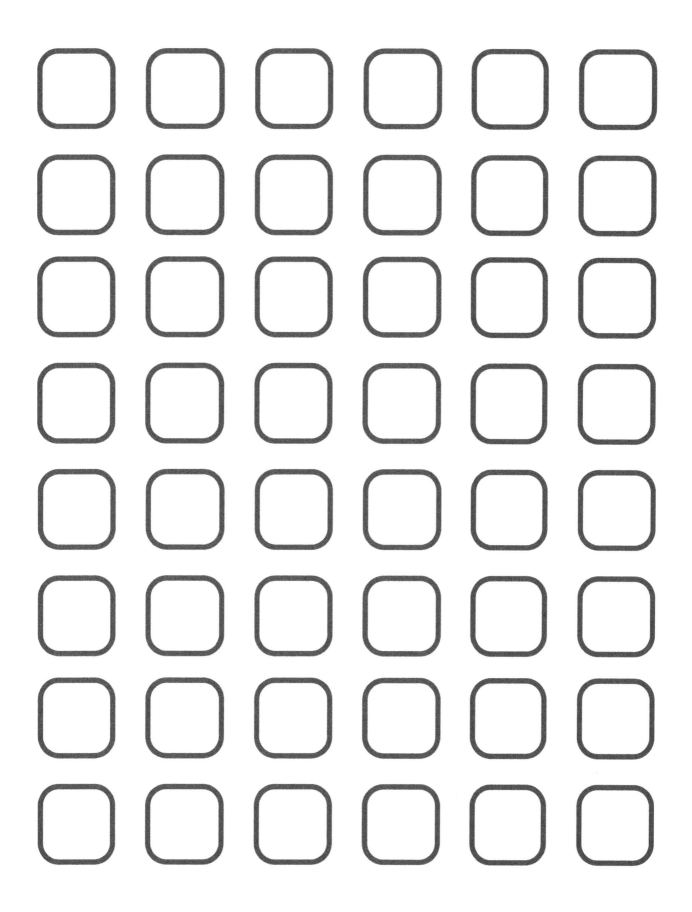

Made in the USA
Columbia, SC
24 June 2024

37353551R00076